9 TIPS ON HOW TO ELIMINATE BELLY FAT AFTER BABY

OLAJUMOKE O. AKINTOLA

ISBN: 9798353399483

DEDICATION

This book is dedicated to my Mum Mrs. S.O Akintola as well as to all of my students, even those who have not yet discovered my contents.

CONTENTS

Terms and Conditions
LEGAL NOTICE

The purpose of this article is to inform you on how to reduce baby fat. Every attempt has been made to ensure the accuracy of this article. Typographical or content errors might exist, though. Additionally, the information in this study on quickly shedding baby weight is only current as of the time of publication. In order to lose baby fat quickly, this report should only be used as a guide.

This report's main goal is to impart knowledge. The author and publisher make no claims that the data in this report is accurate or up to date, and they disclaim all liability for any mistakes or omissions. Regarding any loss or damage caused or purported to have been caused directly or indirectly by this report, the author and publisher disclaim all liability and obligation.

INTRODUCTION

The majority of women struggle to lose abdominal fat after giving birth. New mothers have a lot on their plates between caring for the baby, having sleepless nights, and making future plans. They also need to look after their bodies and minds. Post-baby belly fat is normal, but if it is causing you discomfort, we can assist. Since you may feel that you will never be able to shed belly fat due to your round, squishy stomach, let me explain. But don't worry, you can quickly get back in shape with the correct activities, dietary alterations, and lifestyle adjustments.

See suggestions for reducing belly fat after giving birth. Additionally, we go through ways to get rid of the small bloating that still appears on your stomach. Scroll down!

Exactly why do I still appear pregnant?

These are the causes of why you can still appear to be pregnant.

- Imagining a balloon for your tummy Slowly, your belly stretches as your child grows. The balloon won't pop when your baby finally emerges. The air inside the balloon slowly escapes instead. In addition, despite being compressed and having lost the majority of their air, balloons frequently retain a little amount of air.
- Following delivery, the uterus gradually returns to its pre-pregnancy shape as a result of hormonal changes in the body. However, the uterus doesn't return to its pre-pregnancy size for 6–8 weeks.
- Your body stores the excess food you eat during your pregnancy as fat.

Furthermore, as you are aware, belly fat is difficult to lose and necessitates patience and careful attention.

How long before my stomach returns to its original size?
A new mother's stomach rarely returns to normal in a matter of days. It usually takes a few months for new mothers to return to normal size. Sadly, not all pregnant women manage to get rid of the pouch. Don't worry; if you maintain an active lifestyle, eat wholesome foods, and adhere to a few helpful suggestions, you can easily lose the mother belly. Discover what you should do to lose belly fat after giving birth in the next paragraphs.

Best Strategies For Losing Belly Fat Following Pregnancy

How can I reduce my weight in a healthy way to make my stomach look better?

1. Feed Your Child Breast Milk

Breastfeeding not only helps build your baby's immunity but also helps you lose the baby fat and reduce the post-pregnancy belly.

In the initial months after giving birth, breastfeeding may be beneficial. Though the precise number varies depending on the individual, breastfeeding causes you to burn more calories while producing milk. There's a chance you'll shed your pregnancy weight faster than mothers who give their children formula, but it not assured.

Breastfeeding also causes contractions that cause your womb to contract, which could speed up your weight loss. However, even if you breastfeed, you will gain weight if you consume more calories than you expend.

Losing weight when nursing is acceptable. Your body is quite effective at producing milk, so shedding a few pounds in a week shouldn't have an impact on your production.

But you'll need a lot of energy if you're taking care of a newborn. Soon after giving birth, attempting to lose weight might cause recovery to be delayed and increase fatigue. Avoid attempting a diet with extremely low calorie intake in particular. Hence, attempt to delay your weight loss efforts until after your postnatal check.

You can lose weight by eating healthfully and doing light exercise. You can reach and keep a healthy weight by adhering to the general recommendations below:

- Don't forget to eat breakfast.
- Consume no less than five servings each of fruit and vegetables each day.
- Fill up on foods high in fiber, like oats, beans, grains, lentils, and seeds.
- Every meal should contain a starchy food, such as bread, rice, pasta (ideally whole grain versions for extra fiber), or potatoes.
- Avoid meals like biscuits, cakes, fast food, and takeout that are heavy in fat and sugar.
- Keep an eye on your snack intake between meals as well as your mealtime quantities.

2. Consume Healthy Food

Following childbirth, many women commit the error of missing meals or substituting dietary supplements for a healthy meal. You must maintain your nutrition in order to make enough milk. Micronutrients that support the newborn's body's metabolic cycle and promote healthy postnatal development should be added to it. When doctors and dietitians suggest that you need energy, believe them. To help your body eliminate toxins, fill up on green leafy vegetables, other colorful vegetables, lean protein, spices, green tea, and lots of water.

3. Don't Go On Extreme Diets

Sometimes after giving birth, new mothers experience panic and depression. And in an effort to regain their shape, they engage in excessive behavior and diets that leave them undernourished and ultimately harm the health of the unborn child. Starving yourself won't solve anything; it'll only make things worse. To learn what to eat, how much to eat, and when to eat it, consult a nutritionist.

4. Take A Sleep

You may gain more weight if you don't get enough sleep, did you know that?

Lack of sleep results in a buildup of toxins in the body, which leads to inflammation. The movement of the fat receptors to the center is a result of the body being in a constant state of inflammation. Additionally, the fat molecules are kept in the abdominal area. It can be challenging to get enough rest when there is a newborn in the house, Without sleep, your body is in sympathetic mode all the time.

To put it simply, this indicates that it is constantly accelerating in order to provide the energy required to keep you awake.

High stress levels, increased water retention, and fat accumulation are all linked to this.

Without a doubt, After having birth, you'll probably have sleep issues. even more so if you nurse every two hours.

However, you also need to figure out how to get some rest.
Your stress levels will drop, your energy levels will rise, and sleeping will help your body heal.

Things required to lose weight.

So how do you go about doing this?

- Do not hesitate to take a nap. Throughout the day, take a few naps. If the infant is napping, take a snooze as well.
- Enquire about assistance. One or two of your chores being handled by someone else can help you make time for self-care.
- Make an effort to exercise. According to studies, those who work out frequently have a better night's sleep. Try your best.

5. Exercise

Losing weight and toning your abs are both benefits of exercise. Even in the initial weeks following your baby's birth, you can engage in brief physical activity like walking and stretching.

Start carefully and gradually increase your exercise levels if you were not exercising before to becoming pregnant or are new to fitness.

Regardless of fitness level, all new mothers should start pelvic floor exercises as soon as they feel ready and should work on gradually toning their lower abdominal muscles. Your tummy may flatten as a result, and you may get back to the shape you had before becoming pregnant.

Take your infant for stroller rides whenever you feel up to it. Going outside will make you feel better and give your body a gentle workout.

6. Get Fit

You must get in at least 30 minutes of cardio and weight training if you want to get rid of that stubborn tummy fat you gained after giving birth. Take action when your child is sound sleeping. When your infant is asleep, go for a workout. Perform exercises such as leg raises, jackknifes, tricep extensions, Russian twists, high knees, crunches, push-ups, planks, and spot jogging. However, before you do anything, you should speak with your doctor to find out whether there are certain exercises you should avoid.

7. Meditation Can Help You Relieve Stress

For a few months, you won't be able to do the activities you want to do to help reduce your stress because caring for a newborn baby is highly demanding. Therefore, it is advisable that you engage in meditation as it will aid in improving the quality of your sleep while also allowing you to focus and reduce background noise. The sleep of your infant won't be disturbed, which is the most vital factor.

8. Consider Belly Wraps

Belly wraps or maternity belts may assist you tuck your abs and hasten the uterus's process of shrinking back to its former size, similar to body wraps for total body weight loss. One of the oldest methods of abdominal fat loss is this one. However, studies suggest that belly bands could aid in bettering posture and easing back pain. You need to wrap a soft piece of cloth around your midsection. Verify that it is not excessively tight or loose. But you can also utilize pregnancy belts that are sold in stores. Before wearing the belt or putting a soft cloth around your stomach, see your doctor.

9. Make A Full-Body Massage A Priority

Without needing to work out at the gym, getting a massage can help you lose weight quickly. To help you lose belly fat, have a massage that focuses on your belly. It will help you lose baby fat by releasing and dispersing fat throughout your body and enhancing metabolism. For optimal benefits, have a massage once a week. Even so, further research is required to prove the effectiveness of targeted massage for fat loss, even if there is some data that suggests massage treatment aids in weight loss in obese people.

SUMMARY

Don't start working out right away.

Always start with your diet, then go on to self-care, and last exercise.

Additionally, nursing has a lot of benefits. After giving birth, abdominal fat gradually disappears. Bear in mind that abdominal fat is naturally resistant and that losing it requires patience and work. It will also take some time for your body's hormonal and physical alterations to return to their pre-change states. To efficiently lose belly fat after giving birth, use the strategies stated above. For best results, combine these suggestions with a balanced diet, a healthy way of life, and regular exercise. The weight you added while pregnant will gradually decrease as you apply these tips.

ABOUT THE AUTHOR

Olajumoke O. Akintola is a goal oriented, tireless worker who sees possibilities in all things regardless of the situation. She believes regardless of how many times you fall, try rising again.

What makes this book unique is that you will be able to recognize and take advantage of how to reduce baby fat after giving birth,
Best Strategies For Losing Belly Fat Following Pregnancy,
How can I reduce my weight in a healthy way to make my stomach look better?

www.ingramcontent.com/pod-product-compliance
Lightning Source LLC
LaVergne TN
LVHW052116160826
845678LV00015B/3586

* 9 7 9 8 3 5 3 3 9 9 4 8 3 *